FOOD EXPLORER'S PASSPORT

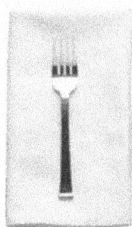

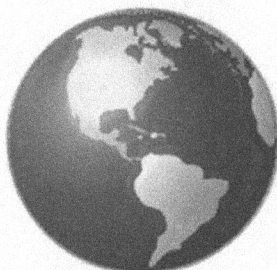

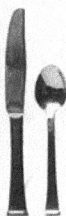

FOR MEALTIME ADVENTURES

Susan L. Roberts, MDiv, OTR/L

Food Explorer's Passport: for Mealtime Adventures

Published by
Element Publishing
Queens, New York 11358

ISBN 978-0-9846847-24

Printed in USA by CreateSpace

How to Use the
Food Explorer's Passport

Let the *Food Explorer's Passport* help you make trying new foods REALLY *exciting and FUN!* Use your *enthusiasm* to encourage children and remember that children and adults have different responsibilities at mealtimes.

Adults have responsibility for **purchasing and preparing foods**. Adults decide **when** and **where to serve** food and they must teach children **how to behave** when eating food with others. Sharing meals together as a family or group helps children grow strong and healthy, emotionally as well as physically.

Children must have control of their own bodies. This means they get to be the *boss* of **whether** to eat or *try* foods using their eyes, fingers, nose, lips, tongue, mouth or teeth. Children also get to be the *boss* of **how much** to eat. Giving children control over their own bodies through these choices empowers them to explore new foods on their own terms, and they grow up feeling strong and whole.

Guidelines for Mealtimes

— STOP fighting about food at mealtimes.

— STOP making your child special meals. Serve one meal to the whole family and let your children choose, from the meal you serve which ones to eat at that mealtime.

— If one of the family needs a special diet, provide foods that meet those dietary needs, rather than cooking a special meal just for that person.

— Serve meals or snacks with 2-4 hours between eating events (for optimal regulation of blood sugar).

— Serve only WATER between meals.

— Include only ONE choice the child likes each time you serve a meal or snack. Bread, rice, pasta and crackers make good choices for family meals. Fruits make good choices at snack time.

— Avoid sugary, sweet foods and beverages. They have very little nutrition to grow your child's body and brain. Children who fill up on *sweets* don't get hungry enough to make healthy choices.

— Put an extra plate or bowl next to your child at the meal. Call this the *TRY BOWL*, where your child can put foods to explore this bowl.

Follow These Simple Steps

1. Talk to your child about being the *boss* of his or her body.

2. Take control of **what** meals and snacks you provide and **when** you serve them. (Stop

asking your child what he or she wants. You already know what they like.)

3. Always serve bread, rice, crackers or some food that your child likes to eat at every meal or snack.

4. Serve foods you or the rest of the family enjoy – even if your child does not eat them yet.

5. Provide a *TRY* bowl where your child can put unfamiliar foods to explore them.

6. Let your child decide how to explore a new food. Make no comments, positive or negative, on their choices.

7. Never mention the *Passport* during mealtimes.

8. After the meal, record how a child explored the foods.

9. Offer to write down foods for the child in the *Passport* or encourage the child to do so – only ONCE – if they don't seem interested, let it go. Try again another day.

10. LET YOUR CHILD EXPLORE FOODS IN THE WAY HE OR SHE CHOOSES, and at a pace that feels comfortable for them.

How to Teach Safe Food Exploration
Using the *Food Explorer's Passport*

Focused Snack

Schedule a regular snack time so that you have plenty of time to enjoy trying new foods as a game. Make it a tea-party, teddy-bear picnic, or pirate's feast. Sometimes siblings or friends can help with the game, and sometimes a picky eater needs your full attention. You will know which works best for your child by trying out both scenarios.

Mealtime Use

Make mealtimes, first and foremost, social times. Avoid getting into struggles about food. You can make a rule that everyone at the table has to *try* every food by allowing them to put a food into a *TRY* bowl and from there decide how they want to explore that food.

ALWAYS LET A CHILD DECIDE HOW THEY WILL EXPLORE the food in their *TRY* bowl. Allow a child to comment or experience the food on their own terms without comment from you.

DON'T TALK ABOUT FOOD unless a child starts the conversation first.

Most people take about twenty repetitions of a new food before they learn to like it. All of us have foods we've tried a million times and still don't like. The *Passport* lets you keep track of how your picky eater uses their senses to *explore* a *new* food and whether he or she learns to like that *new* food. Each page of the Passport takes your child one step closer to comfort with a new food.

Foods I Fed to the Dog

Helps a child tolerate ***looking*** at a food in the same room. Go ahead and act SILLY. Remember scientists always test new things on the lab animals first. Remember to play the game. Reassure your child that he can experience a new food at his own pace. Sometimes "Feed It to the Dog" means take it to the garbage.

Foods I Put on Someone Else's Plate

Continue ***looking*** at a new food by passing it to someone's plate (present or absent, fictional or real). Each interaction with a new food brings a higher level of comfort.

Foods I Touched with My ...

Skin to food contact introduces ***texture*** into your child's experience of a new food. Touching brings the food into "intimate" contact and can be VERY *exciting* (the positive spin on challenging).

Touching food to the elbow and cheek increases the *excitement* level.

Foods I Smelled

Smell activates memory and emotions which directly affect the digestive system. This raises the *excitement*. Asking, "does it smell like something else you remember?" or "where do you feel it – in your head, tummy, chest, throat or somewhere else?" provides a way of processing high voltage emotions (i.e. *excitement*).

Foods I Kissed

Lips have as many nerve endings as our fingers so **touch** and **smell** play a role in "kissing" a food.

Foods I Licked

Tongues have lots of nerve endings that process **touch**. **Taste** buds identify salty, sweet, sour, bitter, spicy and savory.

Foods I Hid on My Plate

Moving the food from the *TRY* bowl to one's plate is a BIG DEAL because it cross-contaminates the other foods. Most of us learned the hiding food trick as children, trying to convince our parents, or teachers that we had eaten a food we didn't put anywhere near our mouth. We squashed the food out flat, scraped it back together in a pile, carved out a *bite*, or tucked it under some lettuce. Teach this **_survival skill_** of pushing food around on a plate and *burying* it under other foods to make it *disappear* before going out in public or attending holiday meals. Friends and relatives will likely forget about a child quietly playing with food, but remember loud complaints, whining or crying.

Foods I Spit into My Napkin

Sometimes a child avoids foods when he or she cannot manage chewing and moving them around in his or her mouth. Make sure your picky eater has good enough oral-motor skills to spit unfamiliar foods quietly into a napkin. Practice spitting dry beans or watermelon seeds outdoors to help your child develop this **_survival skill._** Metal trash can lids make a very satisfying target!

This skill saves a child from fears of having to swallow a food that does not *feel good* in the mouth.

Foods I Can Bite

How does it **_sound_** when chewing?   Some children avoid foods because of the way they sound when chewing them.

How Many Times Can I Chew This Food

The **_sound_** of a food changes the more times we chew it. Children get to discover this when we count how many times they chew a food. Use hash marks or numbers to record the number of chews. Remember to let the child decide how many times they will chew a food.

Foods I Like

Repeated exposure to a food on one's own terms creates comfort. Your child will learn to like **_some_** foods, but **_not all_** of them. None of us likes every food we try.

How to Take this *Passport* "On the Road"

Parents of "picky-eaters" often face community meals with a certain amount of dread. The everyday stress of worrying about nutrition gets magnified wondering if *well-meaning* relatives, friends or even strangers will trigger a *melt-down* by commenting on a child's refusal to eat certain foods. Even the most jovial of families sits with tight lips in shocked silence when a picky-eater gags at unfamiliar sights and smells.

The *Foods I Hid on My Plate* and *Foods I Spit into My Napkin* pages helps your picky eater learn **_survival skills_** to avoid negative experiences with unfamiliar foods and the inevitable *food police* one finds at extended family and community events.

Developing these skills will make you and your child feel more confident with unfamiliar foods in community settings. They will make holiday dinners, restaurants, school cafeterias and family dinners at home more pleasant, relaxed and FUN.

For more ideas about getting children to eat, purchase Susan's book *My Kid Eats Everything: a Journey from Picky to Adventurous Eating.* Available at *Amazon*.

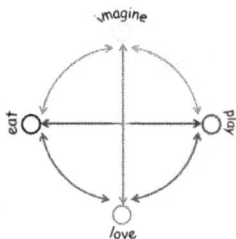

Have Fun.

Play Safely.

Make Friends.

Use Your Imagination.

Foods I Fed to the Dog

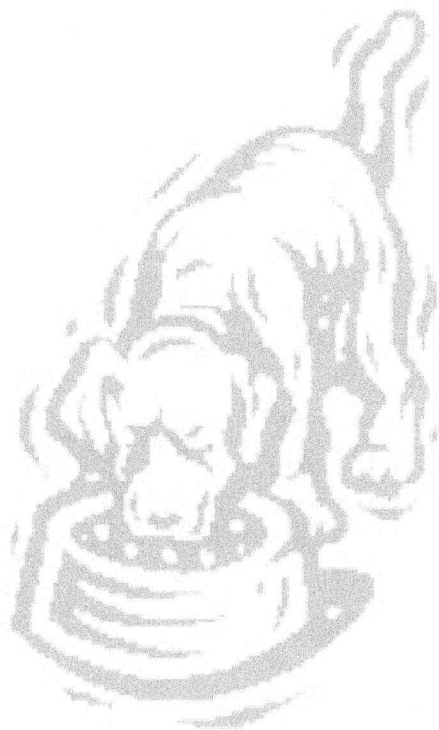

Foods I Put on Someone Else's Plate

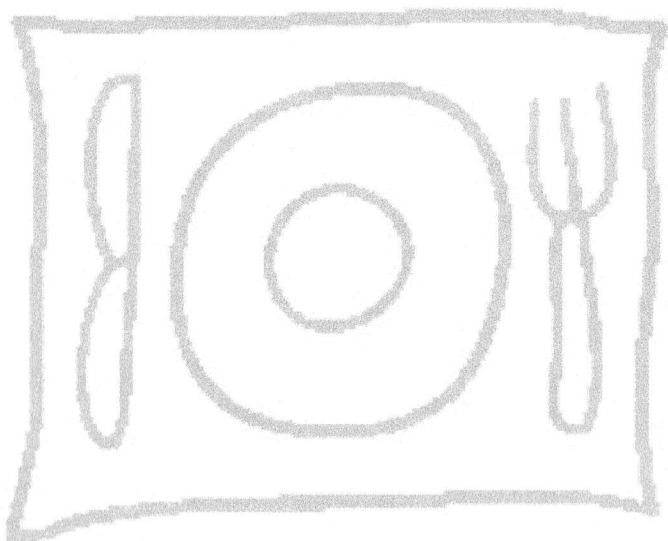

Foods I Touched with My Finger

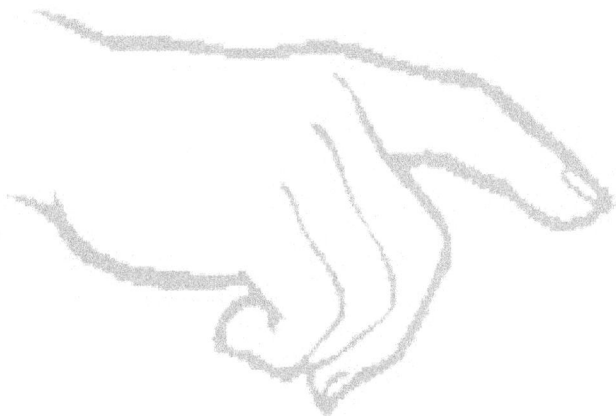

Foods I Touched with My Elbow

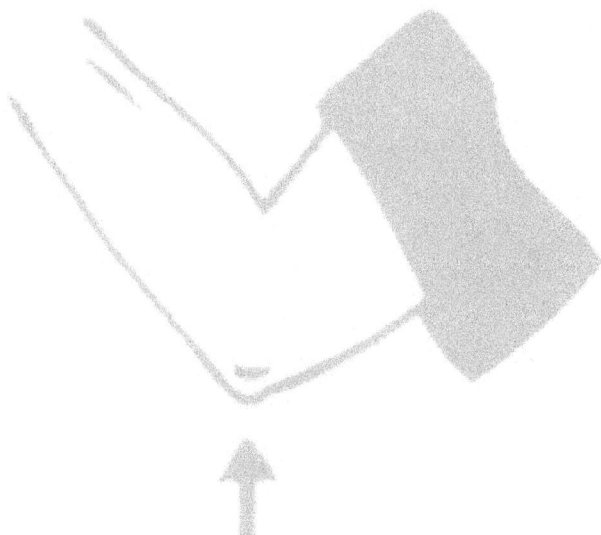

Foods I Touched to
My Cheek

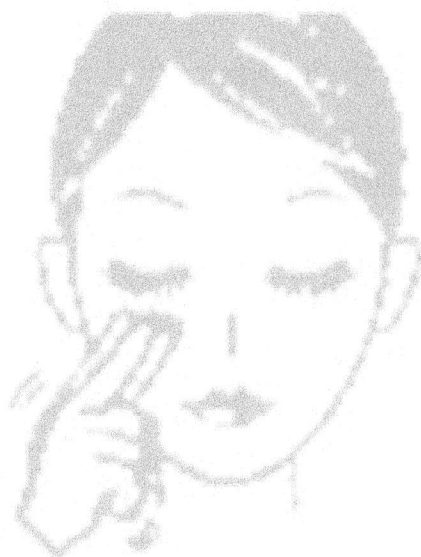

Foods I Smelled

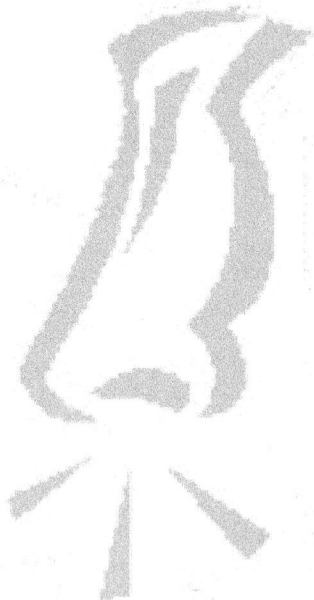

Foods I Kissed

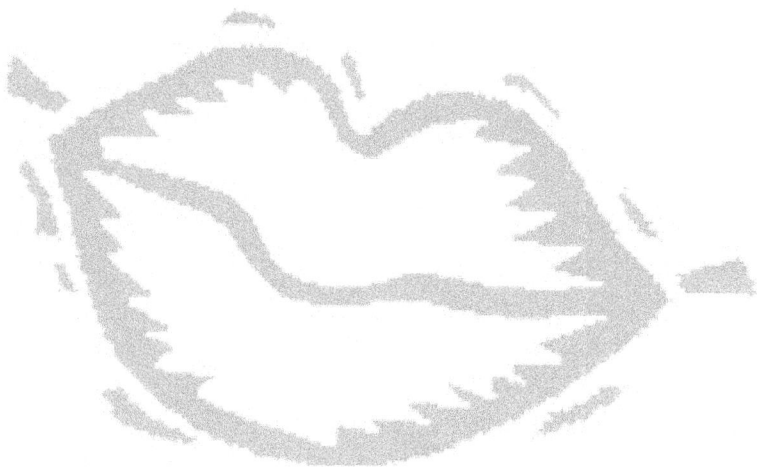

Foods I Licked

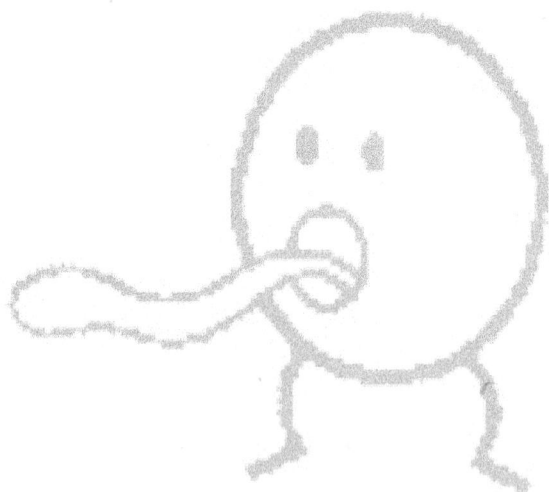

Foods I Hid on My Plate

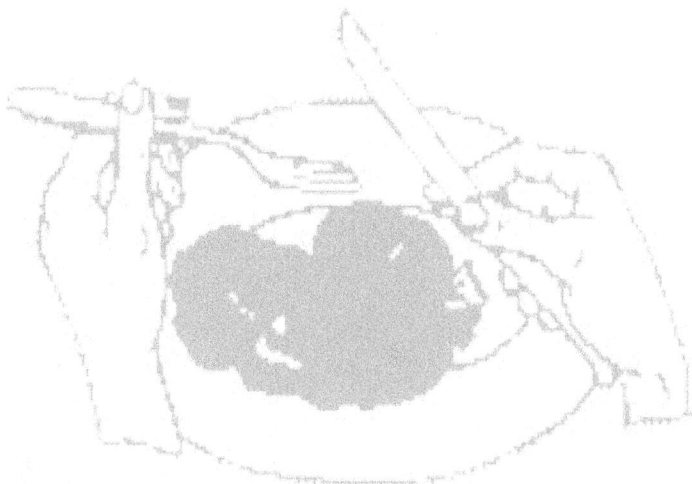

Foods I Spit into
My Napkin

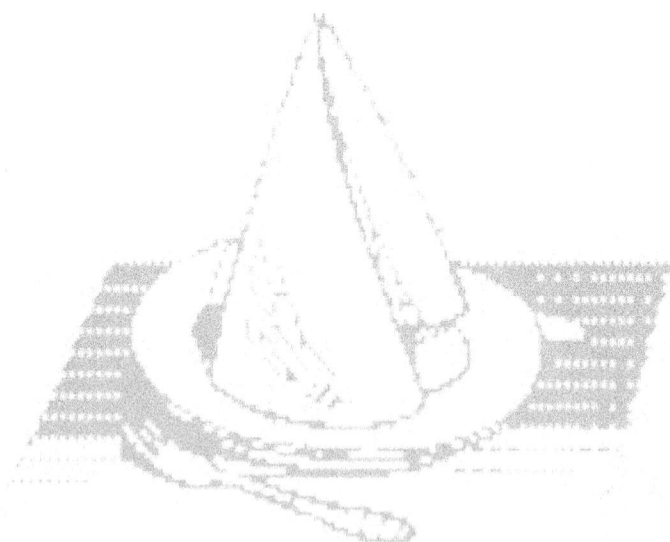

Foods I Put in My Mouth

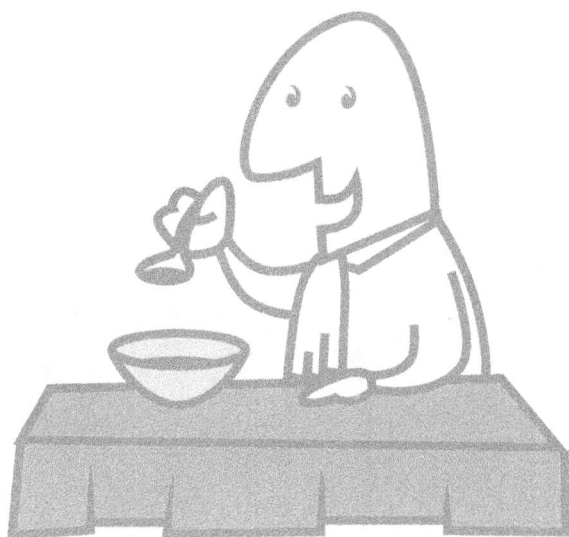

Foods I Can Bite

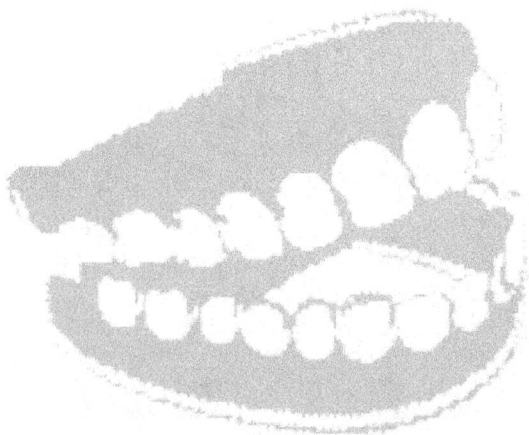

How Many Times Can I Chew These Foods?

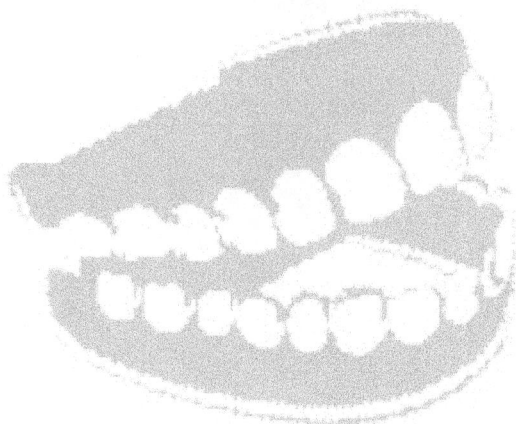

Foods I Like

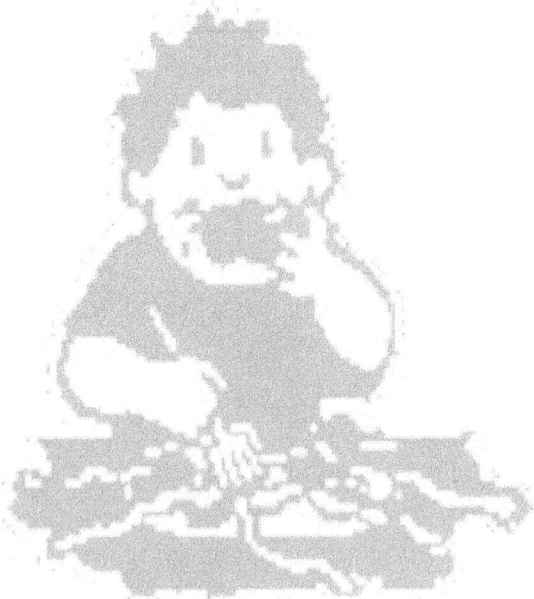

Foods I Like

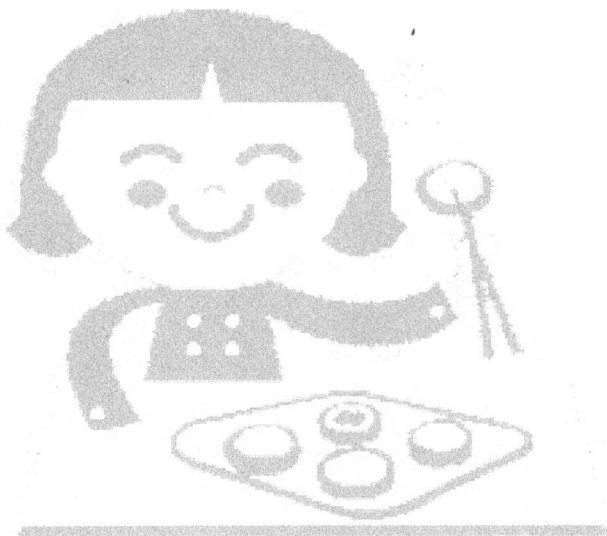